MAF
WILHELMI-BUCHINGER

with the co-operation of
the Buchinger Clinic

Fasting:
The Buchinger Method

SAFFRON WALDEN
THE C. W. DANIEL COMPANY LIMITED

First published in Great Britain by
The C. W. Daniel Company Limited
1 Church Path, Saffron Walden, Essex CB10 1JP, United Kingdom

© Hippokrates Verlag GmbH 1984
English Translation © The C. W. Daniel Company Ltd
1986
Reprinted 1997

ISBN 0 85207 174 4

Originally published in German
under the title, *Die Buchinger-Methode*
by Hippokrates Verlag, Stuttgart

Designed by Tina Dutton
Production in association with Book Production
Consultants, Cambridge
Typeset by Cambridge Photosetting Services in Bembo
Printed and bound by
Hillman Printers (Frome) Ltd, Somerset

Contents

Foreword

The numbers of self-motivated people grow yearly who, by correctly using the fasting methods pioneered by Otto Buchinger, find healing and health. The success of this type of fasting has caused the word to be spread throughout the world. The work of H. Ph. Wilhelmi has contributed to this greatly, and by his own organisation, persuasion and personal initiative he has developed fasting clinics in Über-lingen, Germany and Marbella, Spain. The significance of fasting is growing, not only as a therapy in reducing risk factors involving health, but in the treatment of chronic diseases. As yet it is unknown quite how wide the interest is but there are many books published on the subject and it is well covered on television and radio which must communi-cate to millions, laymen, therapists and doctors alike, the details of fasting. There is a danger, however, of valuable facts being drowned in a flood of advertising and less important information. Because of this, it is essential to use these powerful forms of communication to reiterate the true meaning of this type of therapy and awaken in people the necessity to seek out for themselves practical help. This book is a statement by staff and patients based on decades of their practising the Buchinger Method. It is directed at all those who are aware they have a responsibility for their own health in the context of the community they live in.

It is not possible to rely on the medical skills of doctors alone, nor on any medicines being 'wonder drugs'. Claims cannot be made on the state or health authorities solely to achieve the desired longevity and capacity for both work and leisure. A freely-chosen sacrifice in the form of fasting seems increasingly the safest way of developing a self-discipline that will move us away from a growing chaos of external, and inner, insecurity towards some manageable order. Fasting and the subsequent change in life style remain the fundamental principles we consider will lead to a more healthy and harmonious way by which to live.

The sooner one begins, the greater the success physically, emotionally and mentally. There is no need for illness and injury to be master of our lives, it is far better to prevent illness than to have to find a cure for it. However, it is never too late to adjust and try a new way when perhaps other means have failed.

In effect this book provides the possibility of finding a genuine and truly helpful lifeline for many people.

September 1983   Dr Heinz Fahrner

What is it to be hungry?: what is it to fast?

In the beginning there was hunger

In this book we only touch on hunger briefly, but fasting is dealt with in far greater depth and detail.

We are dealing with two very different terms and so we must be careful not to confuse them.

First of all: What is hunger?
On the one hand
It is a *subjective* feeling controlling the need for food, often this is actually mere appetite for certain foods or even pure craving.
On the other hand
Hunger is actually *objectively* a state of crisis, a plea by the body when it is partly or wholly deprived of food.

How fasting without hunger will develop from hunger

Occasionally, certain disruptions of the general well being and certain pathological conditions will induce a loss of appetite and hence a refusal of food by man and animal alike. As soon as the situation has improved, an animal will start feeding immediately indeed it has to start feeding again; this is not the case with man. He can, if he wants to, fast, that means he can voluntarily decide to forego food for short or longer periods of time. He will then experience that – amazingly – what would have been an agonizing sensation of hunger does not occur.

Freewill

Only man can fast. He will decide to do so by his own volition, and if he does so the organism will adjust to it and arrange to use the reserves of energy stored in the body. Entering into a fast by one's own freewill is of major importance. Therefore, fasting can never be prescribed but only recommended. If fasting is to be devoid of the sensation of hunger and almost completely free from side effects, and lead to positive results then it has to be accompanied by the recognition of the necessity for, and the relevance of, fasting.

Religious traditions associated with fasting

The exceptional results of fasting belong amongst the oldest experiences of man. These have been recorded in the earliest documents of the so-called major religions both of the east and west, Christianity, Islam, Hinduism and Judaism. Fasting in those times was done as a cult and for health reasons. In a fast the person would come to understand how, after the initial changes of mood, tensions would dissolve and a feeling of well being in the soul appear, unknown to him before. In addition those who are gifted in certain ways would often experience astonishing openness towards the principle questions of life or even religious yearnings. At the same time the person will be happy to realise that not only his frame of mind and his spiritual condition were changing in a beneficial way, but against all expectation his physical condition is getting better and better.

Fasting – an ancient method of healing

Moving on from the religious traditions in ancient times we turn to traditions of fasting in those times, or more particularly to the prescription of fasting, when only physical health was concerned, that is when the involvement was with the body rather than the soul.

Throughout the centuries, up to the end of the First World War, fasting was applauded as an effective therapy and a means of 'operating' without recourse to surgery and it was considered the 'King's way of healing' by doctors and laymen alike.

The person fasting had the manner and duration of his fast determined by someone in charge of the treatment. He would rely on the knowledge and insight of such a man to be convinced in all ways as to the circumstances of his fast.

The merit for having developed fasting to the point where it has become a recognised medical treatment with great benefits and without risk to the patient is due to Dr Otto Buchinger. It is for this reason that his name is mentioned in *Brockhaus* and *Reallexikon der Medizin* as 'the creator and teacher of the modern scientifically proven fasting therapy'.

How Dr Buchinger came to fasting

In 1917 during the First World War after suffering from tonsilitis, Dr Buchinger contracted rheumatoid arthritis. This was very severe both in its acute stage and later when it became a chronic condition and as a result his liver was affected. He was, at the time, medical officer in the German marines and had to be invalided out of the service in March 1918 at the age of 40.

His own experience of fasting
Handicapped by severe suffering and restricted mobility, Dr Buchinger managed only with the greatest difficulty to run his general practice which he set up in 1919. Then, a non-medical person advised him to take a fasting cure with

Dr Riedlin of Freiburg. Dr Buchinger said in his autobiography – 'This cure lasted 19 days and almost certainly saved my life and allowed me to work properly once more. I was weak and thin but I could move all my joints again'.

He was still disabled by his chronic liver condition which was accompanied by frequent attacks of gall colic. He undertook another fast of 28 days which completely cured him of these complaints

The man who had been a chronically and severely sick invalid was healed for good; he had not only regained his health but his full capacity to work (and he remained well until his death when he was 89 years old)!

The experience and result of this 'the strongest of all cures' determined Dr Buchinger on his future medical path.

His first fasting patients were introduced to the treatment in 1920 and increasing successes lead to greater numbers seeking this form of help and healing, and they were not disappointed by the results.

Preconditions for successful fasting

Certain fundamental conditions have to be met before a fast can be commenced – as Dr Buchinger recognised from the beginning: The person in charge of the fast must have undertaken several fasts himself.

Successful fasting can only take place where there will be no disturbances. This should be away from the patients normal environment either in a fasting clinic or in a suitable residence with the necessary facilities and experienced staff.

Why fasting should not be undertaken at home
It is inadvisable to fast at home because someone must have medical responsibility for the treatment. There are really no exceptions to this rule except where someone is quite healthy or has already fasted before and is undertaking a short preparatory fast.

Reasons

The reason for not fasting at home is that in not eating one is creating an unusual, even exceptional, situation which can cause greater sensitivity as well as an increased susceptibility to irritation.

Therefore the fasting person has to be shielded from:
— upsets and excitements
— tensions and arguments at work or within the family
— ignorance and a lack of understanding
— a situation where he cannot sleep or rest when he needs to
— temptations
— arguments against fasting
— domestic or other duties

Furthermore the fasting patient must be protected from:
— misinterpretations and wrong assessment of his own possibilities and condition
— bewilderment and insecurity when his general well-being is interrupted
— mood changes which could lead to premature and inappropiate cessation of the fast

The fasting patient needs — and only establishments with experience in fasting can provide:
— an atmosphere explicitly designed for fasting which in itself creates a healing environment
— somewhere sheltered and protected
— security
— distance from everyday life (for which there is already a necessity)
— considered attention

And above all the patient needs an experienced, specialised fasting doctor:
— who determines the length of the fast individually according to the symptoms found on examination
— who is in a position to correctly assess and avert possible crises
— who can, with the support of medically trained assistants and nurses, provide the right guidance and the correct and most important psychological advice at all the different phases of the fast up until it is broken and during the 'building-up' period.

Furthermore, the patient should not be without the supportive therapies mentioned later in the book which act as effective aids to each fasting cure.

Up to 1939 over 10,000 people had undertaken successful fasts on the basis of Dr Buchinger's discoveries and experience. Without wavering he stuck to his firmly held convictions and in consequence the number of beds at Baed Pyrmont Clinic rose to 190.

Fasting is more than losing weight

Estimates made by life assurance companies between the two World Wars calculated that only 7–12% of the general population, and only 2% of the patients in German hospitals, were overweight. From these figures it is reasonable to conclude that the majority of patients in the Pyrmont Buchinger Clinic at that time were of normal or less than normal weight. People came to the Clinic to fast so that they might attain or sustain good health. Remembering that those years, certainly compared with today, were comparatively lean should help to emphasise the real meaning and original value of fasting. However, even those who just want to lose weight will still benefit from the inherent value of the healing qualities of fasting.

Zero Diet

The problems associated with being overweight are some of the biggest in modern medicine. The actual term 'overweight' was unacceptable thirty years ago, but the issue itself has become important because of the disorders accompanying it. These seriously affect the expectancy of practically all age groups, and for the last twenty years various university clinics and hospitals have instituted a drastic fasting cure called the 'zero diet'.

This diet resulted in two specific benefits, in the first place a nil-calorie intake proved the most effective way of reducing weight. In the second, after such a diet, it was found by analysis, that certain body values had been stabilised.

Fasting in Hospital

It should be mentioned here that some people have had unhappy experiences in hospital while on a zero diet because the conditions there are not compatible with fasting. While there, the emphasis was directed entirely at the patient's weight problem, ignoring completely the stimulating effects of fasting. It is interesting in this context to read the report of Britta Graef, when she was in hospital on such a diet.

'I went into hospital to try a zero diet. Although I was perfectly healthy and would have enjoyed some company, conversation and other activities, I was treated as though I were a sick patient.

'Day after day I stayed in a ward full of poor old people who were ill, until late one afternoon when I could bear it no longer I went out. I just walked around, anywhere to get away from the ward and to pass some time. I could not go and sit in a cafe or restaurant. The temptation to eat and drink would have been too great initially, and after a couple of days, when I no longer had any desire for tea or coffee, or even a cigarette, the idea of sitting in such a place all alone was most unappealing.

'I got nothing to eat, just different things to drink; there was mineral water, tea, coffee and a disgusting brew containing vitamins and minerals. It tasted of orange, vanilla or coffee.

'After ten days I could not even stand the sight of it, and smelling or drinking it made me choke.

'Neither the doctors or nurses showed any understanding of my difficulties. They said it was quite simple, and wondered how I could behave so badly, pointing out that my weight problem necessitated this course of action.

'I got no encouraging words, no one came to talk to me helpfully, in fact it appeared that nobody had heard of group therapy or psychotherapy there. They only emphasised that it was all a question of will power.

'The only help the hospital staff offered involved some physical exercises and massages, for the rest it was left entirely to the individual himself. What none of the staff cared to understand was that the patient brings into the hospital not only a weight problem but associated psychological ones as well. These, however, he must keep to himself, for nobody seems to care about them. This, I believe, is why such a high percentage of patients fall back into their old habits.

'During this time my hair became colourless and began to fall out, I got spots on my face and became increasingly tired and depressed. After two weeks I almost suffered kidney failure because I had not had enough to drink, and the uric acid in my blood was double what it should have been.

'At this point I really did become a patient. I had to stop the diet and in its place received special nourishment and pills, added to which the level of uric acid in my blood had to be constantly monitored. So, having fasted for almost three weeks I had lost eleven pounds in weight and had seriously to ask myself if it was worth it.

'The conclusion has to be that the diet did not justify the result and in fact this method of dieting is either no longer used or has been modified. However, any benefits of a zero diet can be achieved quite as well by fasting à la Buchinger while at the same time avoiding its disadvantages.'

The Method of the Buchinger Healing Fast

It is essential that the undertaking of a Buchinger fast is entirely the choice of the individual involved. We consider it of primary importance that a fast is entered into entirely freely, as the element of freewill makes its commencement and course much easier, and the necessary sacrifices possible. Laboratory tests show how the metabolism and the way in which the body functions is affected by the freewill element and the results can be organically proved.

The Fasting Community

To have no fear of fasting but to have a positive attitude towards it, it is best for the patient to be cared for by those experienced in the matter and to be with others who are fasting as well. Such a situation is conducive to a relaxed and friendly atmosphere which is helpful at such an important time. The doctor in charge of those fasting will build up their confidence and make them feel secure. Any doubts or feelings of despair will disappear and such fears will become unimportant.

A Change of Attitude

Before the fast can actually begin, two or three days are set aside so that the rhythm of the patient's routine may be changed. During this time he must become used to his new environment and climate, recover from his journey, and unwind from the stresses of his everyday life. Fasting requires a considerable adjustment so the patient must gradually get used to having no food, or sugar, sweets, alcohol, cigarettes and no stimulants.

A thorough first consultation

Initially the patient will have a thorough check-up with a doctor, laboratory tests will be done and an ECG taken. The results of all these will determine when the patient will begin his fast, how it will proceed and its length.

The length of the fast

The results of the full medical check-up by a doctor will indicate for how long a fast should be undertaken, and the reason for its being a viable treatment. It is necessary sometimes for a compromise to be made as to its duration because of the patients real, or perhaps affected, lack of time.

> The patient can be sure that his clinical fast will only commence once there are no counter-indications. Also the doctor must be certain that the medical conditions exist to, at the very least, ameliorate present problems. The details of his treatment during the fast are planned individually and are subject to the findings of the check-up. In this way the patient sees that he is not being channelled into a rigid fast, but a flexible, personal scheme.

Although each fasting day has its share of success, it must be understood that only a full-length fast produces, for both patient and doctor, a satisfactory result. It has been calculated that at least 21 days fasting with a 6 day building-up period produces the required effect. The length of the fast must not depend on superficial or minor considerations. Once the body has been thoroughly cleansed through fasting then better health and immunity forces should be restored.

In other words, though a compromise may be reached as to the amount of time the patient feels he can spare, it is essential sufficient time is taken for his body to get the maximum benefit from the fast.

The fruit day
The introduction of the fast commences with one to three 'fruit days'. This is a particularly powerful way of eliminating liquids and emptying the intestines, it may, however, be accompanied by headaches which can be quite severe. Patients who have stomach, bowel or gall problems eat natural rice and apple sauce instead; but for those on the fruit diet there is no limit, they may eat as much fruit as they wish.

The salt day
On the first day of the fast, the patient takes 1½oz or 40 grammes of salt (natrium sulphate, which is a salinic laxative) in solution with about a pint of warm water. These particular salts are found in Bertrich, Driburg and Mergentheim.

Although this is not a particularly tasty drink it is quick and thorough. The emptying of the bowels in this way is important because it develops a sense of well-being and relieves the feeling of hunger. The feeling of hunger is also dissipated as the body's metabolism is concentrating on the burning off of existing reserves.

Care of the intestines

During a fast it is most important to take great care of the intestines because a lot of residual matter is being deposited there. The bile resulting from this together with the intestinal bacteria, which normally accounts for one third of the stool, form a mass that cannot be excreted naturally as no food is being eaten. It is, therefore, necessary to help the process in one of the following ways:
    an enema
    or a deeper kind of enema

or another laxative salt drink
or some other laxative prescribed by the doctor
If the bowels are not completely cleared of this residual matter there can be a repoisoning of the system which will noticeably diminish the general physical and mental condition during the fast.

Mealtimes during the fast

It has been proved that it is beneficial to keep a routine during a fast. So after the first salt-day the following regular mealtimes are observed in order to sustain the feeling of a normal day:

---

first thing in the morning
herb teas (there are various kinds, though one in particular may have a specifically therapeutic effect for a certain individual). A cup of black tea or coffee may be required in cases of very low blood pressure or pulse count. A teaspoon of honey is also allowed at this time.
lunchtime
a warm vegetable brew
afternoon
some tea with honey
evening
some fruit juice

Sufficient trace-elements, minerals and vitamins

The vegetable brew for midday consumption is made from a variety of vegetables or potatoes which have been cooked with no salt at all, a little sea salt or some yeast extract. This together with the fruit juice ensures that body is getting sufficient vitamins, minerals and trace-elements to sustain it. Since none of these essentials is missing the patient on a fast feels surprisingly well given the circumstances.

Taking enough liquid

In certain cases, for instance when a patient is extremely overweight, the benefits of the fast can be intensified by omitting the fruit juices, the vegetable brew and the honey and being limited to tea and mineral water. A liquid consumption of about three litres or just over five pints a day is, however, absolutely essential in order that the kidneys, bowels and lungs be thoroughly cleansed. It is easier and there are fewer risks to fasting on 180–200 calories a day. A strict water and tea fast is more difficult but it does give better results.

While the patient drinks the tea and mineral water from a cup or glass, he should actually 'eat' the vegetable brew and the fruit juices using a spoon. It is important that the meals are held in a relaxed atmosphere and at the time one usually has meals. All the patients should eat together and be fully aware of the entire procedure, in this way they will enjoy the simple meals in the company of others.

The daily routine

A typical morning during the fasting period would be as follows:

the doctor's visit
consultations
massages
baths
physical exercises
breathing and spinal gymnastics
training in independence

After lunch, the patient will rest for a while in his room and a nurse will bring him a 'liver-pack'. Because of its cleansing job the liver is under particular pressure and this warm and damp pack encourages its activity. A hot water bottle is provided for the feet as there is a great need for warmth during a fast. The stimulated blood supply to the feet and abdominal area will induce a short but deep and refreshing daytime sleep.

The afternoon programme is likely to involve some of these events:

exercises in the form of:
 walks
 swimming
 water gymnastics
 ball games
 jazz gymnastics
 tennis
 there are courses in painting and modelling etc
 sessions of counselling in the fields of cookery,
 health foods etc
Activities for the evening consist of:
 doctor's lectures (Dr Buchinger called these 'collec-
 tive consultations')
They should give those on a fast helpful and valuable
information and hints gathered from the doctor's experiences with fasting. It should also make clear to patients
what fasting is all about and the way in which their diet
and life style can take a new direction once they have left
the clinic.

Apart from those activities already mentioned there are
facilities for other interests and forms of entertainment, for
instance:

group talks	singing
films	meditation courses
concerts	

All activities at the fasting clinic end at 10 pm or 11 pm
in the summer.

What is taking place in the metabolism during a fast?

The course of the fast

The body needs carbohydrates, proteins and fat in order to function properly. The carbohydrates are sugars which circulate in the blood and are stored in the liver reserves. This supply, however, is fully used up after 24 hours. After that sugar is formed firstly by using particles circulating in the blood, secondly from deposits in tissue and blood vessels and then from old and sick tissue as well as from protein dross. So it is only the lower quality proteins that are being burned up during a fast, while high–value proteins, necessary for tissue building, are preserved. This quite incredible faculty of the body to differentiate between the various qualities of its many metabolic functions helps to control the different metabolism processes in a most significant way. The body rids itself of the poisons it has absorbed; through food, medicines and particularly heavy metals; in a quite determined and specific sequence, and certain rhythm.

The protein question

The need for protein diminishes during the fast until in the second week it has been reduced from 100 grammes to from 15–20 grammes a day, and this amount is in fact quite sufficient while fasting. It is often asked if there are any dangers, or the possibility of damage due to protein loss or deficiency during fasting. This can best be answered with an example. Take a man weighing just over 9½ stone; there is, apart from fat and starch, about 13lb of protein in his body and of that 5½lb is reserve protein,which can be used over a long period of time.

Professor Ditschuneit of the University Clinic of Ulm has written: 'The human body is in a position, because of special regulating mechanisms, to survive complete abstinence from food for many weeks without damaging its health. During a fast the protein loss is reduced to a minimum and strict fasting treatments are effective and carry no risk.' According to research done by the Second Med. Univ. Clinic of Hamburg-Eppendorf, a full fast undertaken without staying in bed and combined with physical exercise does not produce any circulatory problems nor is there any indication of protein loss. It results in no physical weakness and in no way can fasting be compared with chronic under-nourishment or protein deficiency. In the professional magazine *Praxiskurier* it was reported on 7th April 1982: 'Up until now it was thought that those who died of hunger did so because of a lack of protein and that a loss of 50% of protein was believed to be the limit below which death resulted. IRA prisoners who died after 61 days of hunger strike had not in that time used up more than 30% of their protein reserves. It was in fact when the last gramme of fat was burned up that death occurred.'

This remarkable fact can be recognized by another adjustment which takes place in the third week of fasting.

As the fat is increasingly used up it is replaced by substances of particularly high energy combination, this is known as the 'Keton property' which contributes to the saving of sugar and protein already mentioned. The fatty reserves in a person weighing 9st 10lb and 5' 7" tall amounts to about 2st. Two thirds of which corresponds to 93,000 calories in addition to 48,000 calories from protein and carbohydrates. This reserve is enough for about 40 days, a length of time, strangely enough, which has always been considered as the limit for fasts taken for religious or health reasons.

In cases of those who are very overweight it is considered that, under hospital conditions, a fast of 150 or even 250 days is safe. However, such a long fast is considered inadvisable by the Buchinger Method. It is important to stress once again that only a doctor experienced in fasting can advise on the individuals limits and the best length of his fast.

The third week of fasting

Finally, in the third week of fasting the metabolism finds its balance; which is a good reason for continuing the fast for at least this period. With this newly acquired equilibrium comes a feeling of well-being described as 'fasting euphoria', which contrasts strongly with the mental and physical condition experienced in the first days of the fast.

The events described here are considered normal but, of course, there are those who will react differently. In such cases there are clearly definable reasons for the variety of results in patients.

Cases of recurrent illness

Each person has a kind of 'body memory'; it remembers quite precisely disorders which have not been properly taken care of in the past, despite the fact that they may mentally have been long forgotten. So it is possible that symptoms of previous illnesses might appear again; sometimes only as a mere suggestion, much weaker, without so much pain as before and for a shorter length of time.

It is important to observe here the sequence of the symptoms, from acute complaints to illnesses from way back in the past.

Dr Buchinger referred to 'recurrent sickness history'.

However, it does often happen that during a fast health problems, damaged organs or specific physical weaknesses are discovered.

Health during pregnancy

Dr Bircher-Benner, the famous Swiss doctor and founder of a medical diet study, spoke of a healthy pregnancy in this connection. What he was concerned about was that it is possible for a woman to be ill during her pregnancy without noticing or knowing of it. Nothing else highlights this situation as efficiently as fasting. Whether it is a question of an old health problem or one that is discovered during a fast, fasting will influence the present condition of the body as well as cure that which has lingered from the past. There is little doubt that the 'seemingly healthy' pays back his 'illness debts' voluntarily and in instalments. It is possible in this way to prevent an ailment which could strike later perhaps in difficult circumstances leading to a prolonged illness.

Fasting crises

Here are some of the problems which might be encountered during a fast:
— a feeling of being momentarily unwell (this is connected with the strong destruction and elimination of metabolism residue or 'tiring poisons')
— a harmless feeling of vertigo (this is due to a weaker blood supply and distribution which can easily be remedied by light physical exercise, and by moving more slowly, particularly when getting up from either a lying or sitting position).
— having cold hands and feet (this is caused by slight circulatory disturbances which can quite easily be counteracted).
— some sleeping problems (maybe falling asleep, staying asleep or with deep sleep). In these cases natural remedies are most helpful, for instance Kneipp stockings or a light herbal sleeping draught. However, most important of all is the advice given later in the book under the headings 'Television and fasting' and 'Exercise and fasting'.
— the skin breaking out in spots, which rapidly clears up (this occurs because the cleansing process of the fast causes some residual matter to pass through the skin).
— some forgetfulness and a slightly tendency to memory loss (this, too, is part of the same process, in effect the mind is ridding itself of the unimportant and unnecessary things, that which might be irritating or painful is excluded from the memory leaving it less crowded and with space available for good and positive thoughts).

State of health during a fast
If a crisis is sometimes referred to during a fast it is usually a

'healing crisis' which runs its course more easily than might be expected. It may well interrupt the general feeling of well-being experienced by the patient which are characterised in the following ways:
- the capacity of the body for good performance (this is something which makes itself apparent right at the beginning of the fast).
- a more acute sensitivity to environment
- a feeling of greater self-assurance
- a readiness, and enhanced capacity for, meditation

The patient who tries — usually by falsely manipulating personal or business affairs — to shorten the length of his fast, deceives himself and others by trying to outsmart the natural course of events in order to save time.

The fasting body needs time:
- for the repair of residual physical disorders
- for the general, and deep, cleansing process
- for expelling the poisons, fats and liquids accumulated in the body
- for loosening the joints; the circulation of the blood and the tissues cannot arbitrarily decide how to act but must answer the needs of the body (that is the inner organisational principle present in everyone) and the duration of the fasting time must be handled by the doctor.

Short fast:
- means a short lived success
- means taking on only the most difficult, that is the first, days of the fast
- means experiencing only an approximation, of any of the feelings of well-being
- means especially that a repoisoning can be induced once the elimination and process of dispelling the poisons is stopped before the right time. It is for these reasons that it is necessary, almost without exception, to continue fasting even when a 'crisis' occurs.

A long fast particularly one of more than three weeks, or whatever length the doctor judges adequate and necessary, guarantees the best possible results and a good, long–lasting effect.

However, whether it is a short or longer fast you will always obtain a better outcome from fasting than from any other therapeutic method.

One fasting specialist, Dr Zabel, said 'Hardly any other healing method reaches so deeply into a sick body as fasting.'

What can be damaging about fasting?

Though applicable only indirectly, it is worth quoting here from Goethe's *Faust*:

> 'The first one is given us free
> By the second, we have become it's slave.'

Fasting and the meaning of abstinence

Pursuing the Goethe analogy 'the first' is the initial decision to fast; however, the way in which we go about it is 'the second' and in this way we may become the slave of the consequences.

In other words:

When undertaking a fast the patient must understand the implications of 'full abstinence' and have the will-power to forego:

food
tobacco
alcohol

It cannot be over-emphasised that there is no avoiding total adherence to these rules. Dr Buchinger's healing fast would, long ago, have been forgotten, like so many other diets and healing methods, if changes and compromises had been made to the length and discipline of its structure by anyone wishing to do so.

The strict rule of no food

Although it seems quite reasonable not to eat during a fast, it must be stressed that this rule has to be kept most strictly.

The patient must not give in:
— to a passing urge to satisfy his appetite
— to the private thought that 'a little would do no harm'
— to a convincing argument from someone else.

He must remember that:
Each and every morsel has to be digested, throwing the metabolism out of its newly achieved functional mechanism and reversing the effective pursuit which had been successfully begun. This could trigger off a crisis or more unpleasantly something like colic; but worst of all, the patient will feel hungry again, a sensation that would have more or less disappeared after the first days of fasting.

A small quantity of food will excite the appetite without satisfying it. It is for this reason that fasting is a much easier way of losing weight than any other. With the alternative methods there is this feeling of hunger which often causes the patient to give up before he has finished the diet.

Smoking and fasting

It is quite as damaging to smoke when fasting as it is to eat when fasting. Extensive research has established that smoking is a serious threat to our health and it is an equal hazard to fasting. The capillaries begin to shrink after only a few puffs on a cigarette, the blood circulates more slowly and there is partial congestion in the finest arteries, which in fact contribute three quarters of the total of the body's blood vessels (this represents about 75,000 square yards which is almost the size of a football stadium). It takes about an hour for the ill-effects of just one cigarette to disappear. All the organs of the body, and their functions, depend upon a good blood supply and they should be protected from additional burdens like the poisonous tar and cadmium inhaled when smoking cigarettes. The atmosphere is polluted to a greater extent by the smoker with lead and cadmium than the accumulations of a big city.

It has been proved that nicotine is one of the determining factors in heart and circulatory diseases and is irrefutably the main cause of death associated with these illnesses.

The Ministry of Health in West Germany claims that 140,000 people a year die prematurely because of their smoking. Added to this are those 100,000 disabled by smoking. It is calculated that more than twenty cigarettes a day shortens natural life expectancy by twelve years.

Forty percent of all cancers are attributable to smoking and could be avoided by giving the habit up, in the case of lung cancer the percentage rises to ninety. A record number of 2,700 terminal lung cancer cases registered in 1981 highlights the seriousness of the situation.

The British Medical Association has described the cigarette as a 'mass murderer' and the International Health Organisation states that:

'No other factor could save more lives and avoid more illnesses than a drastic diminution of tobacco abuse.'

It would, of course, be much better to say: No smoking at all.

However, all appeals to reasonable usage have been to no effect.

Why fasting is the perfect time to give up smoking

The best time to give up smoking altogether is when you are fasting because the attendant problems of a sudden withdrawal from tobacco are much easier to overcome when there is psychological and medical help. Many heavy smokers are grateful today for their fast because it freed them from this destructive habit.

Sometimes, having just given up smoking, a patient may put on a little weight but this should be considered a small, temporary disadvantage. It is undeniable that a smoker endangers his life to a greater degree than an overweight person.

After considerable research the Medical Clinic of Düsseldorf University considers a man at his ideal weight is thirty percent more likely to die prematurely if he smokes than if he does not.

Alcohol and fasting

The drinking habits of our modern society can produce health problems.

As with smoking, fasting offers the perfect opportunity to give up drinking alcohol. Habitual drinkers can seriously damage such organs as the heart, liver, stomach and bowels and a fast helps eliminate or, at least, ameliorate the harm done.

Not one sip of alcohol

A very strict abstinence from alcohol must be observed. Every glass of wine can either spoil a successful fast or destroy its aims completely. During fasting alcohol can be particularly damaging for the liver. It reaches the blood stream through the mucous membranes in the mouth, the oesophagus and the stomach and when the stomach is empty it is considerably more vulnerable.

Even the first sip of alcohol affects the metabolic functions of the body and can be identified in the following ways:
- it makes all organic activity more difficult
- it irritates the juices in the stomach which stimulates feelings of hunger
- to accommodate the alcohol the system has to use up the body's vitamin reserves
- it has a paralysing effect on a variety of the brains functions
- the performance of the senses is impaired

It appears that some people can take alcohol better than others and differing individual tolerances do exist. However, there is one certainty, and that is whatever the other effects of alcohol, it always damages the health to some degree.

Alcohol is a real poison to the liver

The functions of the liver make it the most important organ in the body's metabolism, and once alcohol is introduced to the system the liver starts the process of 'Burning it off' immediately. A residue is formed as a result which is known chemically as Azetaldehyde and it is a heavy burden for the liver which is accentuated greatly during a fast. The effects are not so detrimental when eating normally but fasting radically alters the situation. In fact the body can be seriously harmed by the alcohol in these circumstances, even in just a short time. During a fast the liver works to eliminate the poisons from the body but if alcohol is drunk it completely blocks this function while concentrating on the alcohol.

The liver can neutralise about 7 grammes of alcohol in an hour, so a quantity of 20 grammes or about a quarter of a litre will occupy it for three hours. So it follows that the more one drinks the longer it takes for the poison to be neutralised, at the same time the alcohol enters the blood stream and steadily rises.

Even once the liver has dealt with the poisoning effects of alcohol the harm can linger on. The cells, for instance, which are damaged by alcohol need longer to recover before they can become fully active again.

Personal Responsibility

Health is not just the responsibility of either the state or doctors, the individual must bear some of it himself. If the patient relinquishes this he dismisses an important element that works toward healing. Professor Petersen of the Medical School in Hanover has forcefully argued against the patient's 'secret wish for medication without a personal effort'.

Given the three indispensable rules of fasting, which are, no eating, no smoking and no alcohol, we can consider this time as an excellent opportunity to acquire new attitudes involving a minimum of self-discipline. To obtain good results from a fast such control will help ensure the patient really gets these maximum benefits. Having this personal responsibility stimulates a new meaning with a practical value.

Various supportive therapies that help the fast

'The far-reaching and wonderful effects of fasting are so basic for me that they do not require further discussion so I can only really view the accompanying care and activities as supportive to the fast.

'However, I must say that without them the treatment would be incomplete. I think that a fast which does not result in the expected success, in spite of the right instruction, is due to the lack of such methods of support.' (*Dr Buchinger*)

Fasting and medicines

When fasting the reactions of the body are different from normal and this fact must be considered by doctors when prescribing either medicines or supportive treatment. During a fast the patient's system is much more sensitive and delicate and reacts a lot more powerfully to all outside stimuli. Any medicines or poisons will cause a stronger effect than would otherwise be expected.

It is important to mention here a specific biological fact. Gentle stimulation assists biological reactions, if it is stronger it blocks these reactions and if far too strong can have a paralysing effect which can eventually cause even greater damage. This rule applies to all physical treatment including air and sun baths.

'The great sensitivity of the patient to medication while fasting allows the prescription of minimal doses of effective substances to obtain the desired result.' (*Dr Fahrner*)

'The art of the doctor lies not only in how to use the necessary medicines but when to dispense with those that are not really required.' (*Prof Hoff*)

When giving treatment, the doctor can eliminate unnecessary medication, retaining only those that are essential; until even they are no longer needed. In certain cases the patient's reactions or metabolism may require his stopping specific medicines or changing to others more suitable.

Allopathy, homoeopathy and other natural healing methods

The doctor concerned will choose whatever type of medicine is most applicable to the patient. He may consider an allopathic remedy from the school of conventional medicine, a homoeopathic one or something from the field of natural medicine. As already established the body is more powerfully affected by outside stimuli during a fast, and will therefore be more receptive to homoeopathic treatment which is what doctors will be most inclined to use.

The homoeopathy of Samuel Hahnemann, for instance, contains no poisons and has no damaging side effects. Such medication is most in tune with fasting and adapted to the faster's body producing good results. Homoeopathic remedies are particularly helpful if a fast is not following its normal course or in cases involving special diseases. 'Also in instances where a fast may have to be interrupted for health reasons homoeopathy allows it to continue.' (*Dr Buchinger*)

'The greatest service rendered by homoeopathy during a fast is not however the healing of a specific illness, which even fasting does not cure, it is much more the fact that it directs the actual fasting process.' (*Dr Buchinger*)

Rödern

To help achieve the correct course for a fast and in so doing avoid any disorders, a stimulating therapy called 'Rödern' (after Dr Rödern of Wuppertal) is recommended.

This particular therapy involves pumping out the tonsils, which are the organs designed to release the lymph in the body. By this action any residual matter is removed reducing the risk of infection, which as with the teeth, can spread alarmingly.

The process also comprises massaging the tonsils and the lower nasal mucous membrane with a soft probe. In turn the hypophyse or pituitary gland, which influences the hormonal balance of the body, is stimulated, and that part of our central nervous system not commanded by will is quite probably affected at the same time. In turn then our breathing, the circulation of our blood, the retention of liquid, the regulation of warmth and our sleeping rhythm are all refreshed.

After many years of experience Dr Buchinger considered the influence of the Rödern therapy indispensable. He said:

'Patients who do not undergo the Rödern treatment have a more difficult fast, in some cases substantially so.'

Massages, packs and water therapy

Although it may be considered rather simple, special massages and water therapy while fasting are helpful and give good results. One of the most desired effects of massage is the increased blood supply not only in the skin but in the tissues and muscles. The circulation of the blood is improved helping the elimination process of the fast and the metabolism is stimulated.

There is a direct correlation between the blood supply and the condition of the skin. When the blood supply is increased the internal organs perform better and the skin looks and feels better.

On the other hand, special skin massages can benefit specific 'disorder zones'. Because manual therapy has such possibilities and effective results, it plays an important supportive role in fasting.

By stimulating the skin, water therapy can influence the condition of the internal organs.

It is possible to stimulate the skin just by changes of temperature with the result that deep-seated tissue and organs have a better blood supply.

Specifically planned therapeutic programmes can include various hydrotherapies from Kneipp-washups, packs, water gushes through to medical baths. These are particularly compatible and supportive in their long-term therapeutic effect.

Sunbathing

The Arndt-Schulz rule relating to the severity of physical therapies is especially valid during a fast in connection with sunbathing and the use of sun lamps.

The idea that 'the more sunshine, the better one's health' is false. Many people sunbathe far too much in order to get a fashionable tan.

It is certainly true that, when correctly used, the sun has healing properties, for instance with rickets, bone- and articular tuberculosis though, of course, such diseases are rarely found today.

However, it is only in small quantities that the ultra-violet rays can be considered medically beneficial so doctors can only responsibly recommend sunbathing for short periods. Damage, either at the time or appearing later, will occur if this rule is ignored and in the short-term can result in:
— either slight or bad sunburn caused by over-pigmentation
— limited or more general insomnia
— attacks of nervousness

It is important to avoid these particularly during a fast. The more long-term damage incurred from repeated over-exposure to the sun are:
— premature ageing of the skin due to its dryness
— the loss of elasticity and greater stiffening of the skin which is conducive to skin cancer
— the loss of red cells

The fact that one is used to long and intensive sunbathing without suffering any special reaction does not preclude damage or resultant complaints manifesting themselves later.

It should not be forgotten that even in the shade fifty percent of the ultra-violet rays reach those uncovered parts of the body. The sun's reflective strength is greatest on the beach, on water and in the snow particularly high in the mountains.

Breathing

Breathing is the most crucial function of the body and due attention should be given to it when fasting.

Bad breathing habits and incorrect breathing movements together with poor posture prevent proper respiration. Well regulated breathing is necessary to facilitate the quite natural and continuous exchange of gases in the lungs. One common misconception lies in the belief that breathing deeply in and out is an important and beneficial factor.

In fact, if more air is inhaled than is really necessary the conditions for taking in oxygen and getting rid of carbon dioxide deteriorate. It is also damaging to force air out as this causes excess pressure which will obstruct the blood supply and hinder the circulation causing further problems.

Breathing is a natural function from the first newborn cry to the last dying sigh, it reacts to all the movements of the body as well as to the fluctuations in the state of mind.

Breathing gymnastics

We have established that it is important to exercise not the breathing itself but
- the organs associated with breathing
- those muscles directly or indirectly associated with our breathing
- the elasticity of the thorax, trunk and diaphragm
- to find the right posture

To inhale more air, natural ways should be used to deepen the breathing by moving, stretching and extending the muscles. Once the muscles are extended impulses will cause corresponding reactions in the lungs. Such extension will be generated by stretching postures used in exercises during breathing therapy, and termed 'organ gymnastics', which are comparable to certain yoga positions.

The results will be a diminution of breathing problems and the correction of poor posture.

It is true to say that it is best just to let the breath come:

The breathing gymnastics involve two methods, one

where the breathing is in unison with the body and the other in which the body works on the breathing. The first technique is conducive to the body taking a full, body-filling breath, and the second involves modifications in breathing.

Taking a full breath is not some technical achievement involving a physical action: 'It occurs spontaneously when the body shows the least opposition or reaches a point when there is the greatest lack of hindrance.' (*Herbert Fritsche*)

There is, however, no substitute for physical exercise in the fresh air, not even the best breathing therapy. It is only with movement that vigorous breathing occurs building up better oxygen reserves.

Physical exercise: an active way of helping

Physical exercise is not only one of a number of therapies used during a fast, it is an active way of helping its progress.

Physical exercise has the most powerful effect on breathing, the circulation of the blood, and the metabolism, and its positive influence is significant in the successful treatment of a fast.

Fasting does not diminish the body's capacity or performance, in fact physical activity is encouraged while fasting. After only a few days of a fast movement and physical effort become easier while the patient's endurance grows and a positive enjoyment of movement becomes evident. Such feelings and impressions related to fasting agree with scientific tests, for instance those resulting from the use of apparatus atttached to exercise bicycles and from ECG's.

It is not possible to save energy during a fast by preserving it. On the contrary it will demand proportionally as much energy as it has avoided using by either forced or unforced immobility

An old biological adage says – the condition and the quality of function of any organ will be greatly determined by the degree and way in which we challenge it.

The disadvantages of too little exercise

If a man is using only a quarter of his muscle ability and just a half of his potential blood circulation he will be deemed as not using or exercising his muscles sufficiently. Not getting enough exercise results in a variety of problems. These include disorders in the function of muscles when atrophy may develop, as well as a diminution in their capacity. The speed at which this can happen is indicated by the thirty percent loss of strength in a muscle after only eight days in a plaster cast.

The movement should never be kept so limited as to only keep the muscle alive. As a rule the organs of the body need a great deal of challenging to keep them functioning not only in good order but also to improve their performance.

According to his build and development a man should use his capacity for movement to the maximum. Ninety-nine percent of man's working energy has been replaced and taken over by machinery now, while one percent is still required by human muscular energy. Our exercise generally revolves around short walks, window-shopping, maybe an hour's housework, and we sit at our jobs, in our cars and watching television. During a fast this degree of inactivity is quite inadequate.

The heart is a muscle and needs exercise

The heart suffers quite particularly from a lack of exercise. Just as an under-used arm or leg muscle will contract because the blood circulation is poor giving insufficient oxygen, so the heart can suffer in the same way subsequently getting smaller and weaker. The heart will in fact reach a state of atrophy just as any other untrained muscle in the body.

The rhythm of its muscular action will develop irregularities, the blood vessels will narrow and the circulation of the blood will be poor. A greater demand for oxygen will evolve but the actual amount available decreases. At the same time the ability of the blood to absorb oxygen is limited so the oxygen inhaled will not be fully used. All this causes the heart to work harder because without physical exercise the blood is not being pumped properly round the body.

The lack of sufficient exercise is now considered as one of the most serious contributary factors to the ever-rising numbers of people suffering heart and circulatory diseases. After smoking, high cholesterol levels and high blood pressure, insufficient physical exertion is the most important cause resulting in complaints associated with the heart.

The combination of exercising and fasting is the ideal way to correct the imbalance induced by inertia on the one hand and over-eating on the other. The excesses stored in the body will be burned off while fasting and the reserves will be used up and developed further.

Overeating + no exercise = overweight

Overeating combined with too little exercise results in a person becoming overweight. If we eat more than is required by our bodies to function efficiently and then fail to take physical exercise, the extra nourishment will cause a build up of fat; such facts do not need to be proved or explained further. Only a few cases can claim that a weight problem is due to hereditary factors, a slow metabolic rate or a thyroid deficiency. In fact it has been tested and proven that thyroid problems cannot be blamed for obesity and do not influence weight problems in fat people.

Obesity and gland disorders

Fat does in fact affect a variety of glands. Overweight people work off fat, carbohydrates and proteins in exactly the same way as those who weigh less. There is really no such thing as a good use for excess fat, it is just a source of energy that is stored as fatty tissue whose only advantage is in fact as a form of insulation against the cold influencing the loss of body warmth. Those of normal weight with no insulating fat lose heat all the time and must replace it by burning energy to sustain the necessary body temperature of 36.5° Celsius.

How do we measure what is overweight?

When someone weights 10–20% over what is considered the maximum desirable they are regarded as being overweight. Once this has exceeded 20% it is called obesity.

To calculate this maximum desirable weight you can take your height in centimetres and subtract 100 to get the answer in kilos. An alternative method, which takes into account your build, is to multiply your height by the measurement of your midthorax, again in centimetres, then divide the answer by 240 and again your weight will be in kilos.

'Ideal weights'

The ideal is the maximum desirable weight less 10% for a man and less 15% for a woman. One person out of three who consults a doctor today is more than 20% overweight. As a rule such a degree of fat has a damaging effect on the health and the extra load will have harmed the heart and the circulatory system of the blood. There is a risk of high blood pressure, a high fat and sugar content in the blood, breathing difficulties and a lack of oxygen getting to the muscles, the tissues and the raised diaphragm. A considerable weight loss is strongly recommended should any of these symptoms manifest themselves.

Losing weight without exercising

Let us look at the possibility of losing weight during a fast without taking physical exercise.

> It is in fact possible to lose weight without much activity but the reduction involves 'lean' not 'fatty' weight. In this case there is a far greater protein loss and some muscular degeneration.

Comparative clinical tests show successful therapeutic results from fasting in conjunction with physical exercise. In such cases the weight loss only affected the fatty tissue without harming muscles.

There is twice the oxygen requirement needed for burning up fat than is used for carbohydrates or protein. For instance one kilo of carbohydrates or protein needs 900 cubic centimetres of oxygen for the burning up process, while 2000 cubic centimetres is required for the equivalent weight in fat. It is only by exercising that the body can absorb this extra oxygen.

It is a misconception that there is no correlation between losing weight and taking exercise. Each movement we make, however small, costs energy, which during a fast is manufactured by burning up existing substances in the body. If one were to walk for an hour something like 300 calories would be used up, depending on how quickly, and on what sort of terrain one walked.

The more one moves the more calories are used up

To make a more precise calculation: if one were to take a walk of say 3 km or 1.8 miles one would work off 220 calories in body weight an hour, if it were 6 km or 3.7 miles then the reduction would be in the order of 370 calories an hour. The calorific need rises with the degree of difficulty involved with the activity or sport. At the same time the increased inhalation of air provides more oxygen, improving the supply of blood to the heart and the entire body.

The figures mentioned above only involve what is used up during an **activity** and does not take into account the active burning up of more calories after the exercise. The metabolic rate is significantly increased after exercise, the effect of which can last some hours, even days when compared with a body lacking such activity.

Sometimes, in spite of exercise, the weight reduction can be less during a fast than previously experienced. The **explanation** for this is that untrained muscle will tire quickly activating a process called 'trans-animalisation'. This involves the kalium in the cells being replaced by natrium which attracts water. In this case the water retained will cause the swollen cells to be heavier. However, the body self-regulates this situation quite quickly and the balance of water held in the body is soon re-established.

We must emphasise that physical exercise is essential to satisfactory weight loss during a fast, because it keeps the muscles in good shape and eliminates, by burning them up, superfluous substances in the body.

It is also through regular exercise, together with a healthy diet that once the fast is over its success can be maintained. Exercise is the essential requirement of all therapies concerned with obesity because as Professor Björn Torp of Göteborg once said 'being overweight is clearly related to a lack of movement.'

Should we exercise?

The expansion of the metabolism and the invigoration of the blood supply activated by physical exercise challenges the heart and strengthens the body. It is, however, necessary for this exercise to be quite vigorous and to extend for some time. Ideally three times a day the pulse should reach 100–130 beats a minute and should be sustained at this level for from 3–10 minutes. This can be achieved by walking on the spot, skipping or walking upstairs.

What is important is higher pulse rate. For older people a reasonable maximum can be calculated by subtracting their age from 180. In this way 50% of the optimum circulation is achieved.

Pulse control

Everyone can control his own heart rate whether it has been overtaxed or remains within its own capacity. Even a small effort which stimulates the pulse can improve the function of the heart by 10% after only one month. This is not very much but could be sufficient to prevent a possible heart attack or heart failure.

It is important to stress the importance of exercise while fasting.

Increasing stamina

Improving the stamina during a fast should be done gradually. Initially it should not be too intensive or too fast, nor should it go on for too long or be excessively challenging. Overall the building up process must activate the whole body.

Active sweating

The training should not cause a loss of breath but stimulate an active breathing rhythm. The skin temperature will rise as the body becomes warmer and sweating will occur which is both welcome and helpful. Sweating in these conditions is different from the passive perspiration experienced when sunbathing or taking a sauna because it results from body activity and releases poisons from the body through the pores of the skin. Such poisons accumulate in the connective tissue absorbed from the environment around us and formed as a deposit of the metabolic process.

It is now accepted that lead, amongst other heavy metals, damages vesicular breathing, and it is believed that this can be cancer inducive. There is proof that 18% more of these heavy metals is released from the body in sweat than in urine.

Apart from this it is interesting to note that the water retaining salt, natrium is discharged in higher concentration in sweat than calcium, kalium and magnesium. This means that less of the more valuable minerals is lost than during more passive sweating according to research carried out at the Institute of Stuttgart-Oberjesingen.

Increased physical exercise does not make you feel more hungry either during a fast or after it. On the contrary whether it be at the 'building-up' stage or later at home it actually helps adapt the body to a diet meeting its real needs.

Physical exercise is particularly helpful to fasting in the following ways:
- reducing the high fat content in the blood serum
- raising the protective blood fats before a heart attack
- improving the hearts function while diminishing its effort
- reducing high blood pressure
- improving the circulation in the small blood vessels of the legs and in the area of the heart, and building new blood vessels around the heart
- making better use of the oxygen in the body

– increasing the breathing capability by a thorough airing of the lungs
– multiplying and enlarging important cell components in the muscles
– causing the burning up of fatty acids in the muscles
– relaxing tension and cramp in muscles
– strengthening weak muscles by releasing tension
– reducing the body's insulin needs
– inducing longer and more restful sleep
– helping to create a happier general state of mind
– giving a new zest for life.

A 60 year old man who regularly exercises is fitter than one of 40 years who takes no physical exercise. It is, of course, true that one cannot actually become younger by exercising but it is possible to retain the fitness of a 20 year old.

It is quite unnecessary to have concern for any disadvantages resulting from sports, one should be much more inclined to worry about a lifestyle devoid of physical activity.

Walking

Walking is a form of exercise available to everyone and can be done regularly everyday with the minimum of effort. Starting with a quite slow and easy style of walking then the transition to a more lively and quick walk can be fairly gradual.

Long walks

Irrespective of the season or the weather, long walks are a central part of the exercise programmes arranged during a fast. Routes are devised with varying degrees of difficulty involving some climbing as this is considered more therapeutic than walking on flat terrain. As you walk it is important to breathe through your nose and it is best not to talk particularly when going up hill as this tends to disturb the rhythm of the heart and breathing.

Interval training

It is quite effective to use the so-called 'interval training' on an excursion into a hilly or mountainous area. The changes involved in going either up or down hill, or alternatively taking 190 fast steps followed by 200 slower ones, forces the circulation to adapt itself to the variations. This helps combat circulatory disorders particularly in the legs much more successfully than with the use of medicines.

Bicycle rides

Bicycle riding is a further exercise available should there be insufficient weight loss or if the joints remain arthritic.

Swimming

Swimming is quite the best form of exercise for anyone suffering from asthma. It is an excellent form of physical activity as it makes the whole body work without overburdening it.

Modern gymnastics

In an attempt to find a form of exercise that uses the entire body evenly modern gymnastics evolved, as found, for instance in the School of Hinrich Medau. They are characterised by the following type of activity:

walking, running, bending, jumping and swinging performed with or without such equipment as a ball, rope or loops.

The basic forms of gymnastic activity answer the natural requirements, potential and instincts we all possess for exercise. When accompanied by music and the rhythmic and harmonious movement of the body and mood exercises gives a feeling of total accord.

Dancing

Dancing is a pleasant and undemanding form of exercise. 'It is not regarded as needing much effort and consequently you exercise without noticing it and forget entirely that you are doing something which is good for your health.'

It particularly enables older people to rediscover and manage their bodies, dancing in a group, in pairs or simply alone. It is understandable that a patient who is overweight should feel a little self-conscious and be unwilling to participate but he should forget his embarrassment and force himself to join in and not just to sit and watch.

'When dancing, even alone, one can become an equal member of a group by introducing any variety of actions and sequence of movements. It is impossible to appraise the amount of energy expended while dancing, particularly during a fast but there is a special bonus to this sort of exercise, and that is how enriching it is for the soul.

'Exercising and fasting are essentials for man in this technically developed world.'

The state of our soul while fasting

Already discussed are a number of helpful therapies, however, 'there is still a very important one, if not the most important one, which should be included in all treatments but is especially relevant to fasting.'

Soul healing therapy

'By this we mean guiding the soul, the healing soul therapy.' (*Dr Buchinger*)

Though different languages have other ways of saying it, it comes down to the same thing. It may be approached through psychotherapy or with psychosomatic medicines or by other more general methods, we call it 'soul healing therapy'. Whatever the course taken, the aim of the treatments is the same.

The deeper value of a fast, its fundamental purpose, lies in its influence on the soul and the spiritual side of the patient.

Even when at the beginning the faster's thoughts still linger on food, as well as matters concerned with his health, he will desire or perhaps more accurately his soul will desire some solutions which will carry him beyond just a weight loss or the cessation of pain. Fasting is an all-embracing treatment affecting both the body and soul, and at the same time it is both appealing and challenging.

Fasting is a time for looking back and thinking things

over in terms of assessing possible changes in one's way of life. But to achieve a healthy state of mind and soul one must start with the body
- by separating the good elements from the bad
- by making sacrifices in terms of excitement and distractions
- by the handling of irritations and problems

Television and fasting

The effect of watching television should be seriously considered as a stress factor in our lives and account taken of the damage it might do to someone fasting.

After much research the medical findings indicated that watching too much television resulted in headaches, extreme fatigue, an overloading of the vegetative nervous system, an over-active feeling of fear, sleeping problems, a rise in heart frequency and diastolic blood pressure, a disturbance of the heart's rhythm, and too little physical activity.

The assault on the brain is twice as great from optical stimulation as from acoustic impulses and the effect only recedes after some hours when it allows only a somewhat troubled sleep level to be found. People often have problems sleeping after watching television. It also diminishes vitality and leaves the brain less receptive while there is a falling off of concentration and a lack of stamina producing sudden fatigue.

For an improvement in such conditions it is advised that there should be no television for from two to four weeks. Television over-burdens the eyes forcing them constantly to adapt to changing images, something which will eventually damage their capacity for adjustment.

In addition to this it would be well to take account of what we are actually watching, albeit sometimes for only short periods. It is worth considering the cleansing effects to the soul a period of abstinence from television would bring. That is why, during a fast, which after all is designed to bring health to both body and soul, we strongly recommend that watching television is avoided.

Fasting atmosphere

To derive the greatest benefit from a fast it should be undertaken in a special atmosphere, a special climate. It is possible that once we are free from what restricts our senses and our souls we can 'hear' and appreciate the silence. It is an important factor in fasting, this:

Silence

We never take the time to reflect upon it, or do so far too rarely.

Silence, to get back to oneself

Marc Aurel said: 'You are free at any time to go back into yourself. Give yourself this right often, and return back into yourself and you will become younger.'

It is, however, in our everyday lives that we do not find the necessary silence because we are constantly distracted and nervous we often ignore the importance of quietness.

'In returning, and rest you shall be saved, in quietness and in confidence shall be your strength; and you would not.' (Isaiah Ch 30 v 15)

Meditation

Should we try to be quiet while fasting?

Meditation can assist us in this respect.

To describe meditation one uses many words – contemplation, reflection, introspection, thinking about a symbol or God; letting oneself drift away mentally without any fixed aim, listening within oneself; self realisation, a closeness to God or simply striving for a balance between body and mind.

There are many forms of meditation.

Today the most popular forms of meditation originate from the Orient probably because they seem best able to answer the needs of our time. However, it is questionable whether a form of meditation combined with a hindu or buddhist teaching of self-deliverance should be accepted without some criticism.

The India expert, Ernst Gogler, warns that following an oriental meditation technique really requires the services of a guru to help control the overwhelming pictures and thoughts that are experienced.

It is a mistake too, to assume that forms of meditation come only from the East.

'In the past there existed many Christian ways of meditating which served to strengthen faith and heal the soul.' (*Alfons Rosenberg*)

Autogenous training or Self-generating meditation

The most helpful form of meditation while fasting, is the autogenous or self-generating method. It is also beneficial in finding one's own way. The Germans express it as 'exercising which comes from the soul'. However, with this method as with the others it is important that an experienced teacher is on hand during this 'concentrated self-relaxation'.

Psychotherapy

Fasting cures should always be complemented by a course of cautious, well-directed psychotherapy.

Talking is the basis of all psychotherapy and during a fast the conditions are particularly favourable. Dr Buchinger said, 'Fasting frees and relaxes the mind and soul and offers them for communication'.

'There is plenty of time available while fasting, much more than under normal hospital and consulting room conditions. When not attending other therapies, the fasting patient can use his spare time to get problems off his chest with his talking partner without fear of disturbance or being influenced by questions, in fact in complete freedom.

'The doctor involved will have a mixture of expectation and reservation, he will not press for a quick result from his therapy. He, too, has plenty of time and can wait for the desired result of the therapeutic fast.

'The doctor–patient relationship really profits from the wide time span involved in a fast. The bond which is important to good results in psychotherapy, has sufficient time to develop.' (*Dr Winckler*, Munich)

Problems concerned with health which so often have associated psychological conflicts and opposing background situations can be recognised and worked on.

There is the time to discover misjudged attitudes and communication difficulties, as well as a chance to look at one's view of oneself and others and if necessary and desirable to change them. Reassessed attitudes taking the place of dissatisfaction, frustration, impatience and an exaggerated ego will accelerate the healing process and prepare the way for lasting good health.

We can quite easily acknowledge the existence of all the contrasts in our world; light and shade, health and disease, and happiness and unhappiness. To make it possible to alter what we are able to change we must first have the strength to cope with what is inevitable and unchangeable.

Fasting and religion

The strength we have just mentioned can grow out of faith or through prayer. Dr Buchinger became aware of this early in his career and commented 'The world of prayer – in fact in religions generally – and the world of fasting are closely related. Indeed, each one promotes the other. It is here that the religious aspects of any fast should be apparent in the mind of the supervising doctor, to help in the care of the soul. He should introduce it into his treatment with as much tact, caution and competence as he can. This very special and beautiful practice is mentioned in a book called 'Das Heilfasten' but still it belongs to a somewhat mysterious and unspoken domain. The fasting specialist is required to concentrate on the most profound aspect of the patient so that he can address himself to the surge of spiritual need surfacing during the fast. All this is what I have learned after forty years of treating fasting men and women.'

The small psychotherapy
Goethe has provided us with a simple recipe for a more

compact therapy to enrich our lives, give us strength and help us to regain the equilibrium of our souls: 'Each day one should listen to a beautiful song, read a lovely poem, see a fine painting and when possible speak a few words of wisdom.'

Reading as a therapy

It is important that the fasting patient should read; for now he can study books without being disturbed. The concept of 'biblio-therapy' contains the idea that literature itself can be therapeutic, it can bring consolation and strengthen hopes. From poetry, man acquires symbols, it is an ambassador of his thoughts.

Music – medicine for the soul

Music, too, contains a consoling and healing power. This I realise is a rather poor description of what since ancient times has been accepted as the great healing effect of music. Plato said: 'Music is a medicine for the soul.' Music has, in fact, long been used therapeutically to treat disorders of the mind and associated organic problems.

'Rhythm, sound and melody influence changes in the minds and bodies of mankind. What could be better than introducing music into the diet of the inner-man paricularly during a fast.' (*Dr Buchinger*)

We are really lucky today because there are such musical treasures to be found which are easily available; they have only to be unveiled.

Fasting makes people more receptive, they are more open and respond to positive and negative impressions readily.

Overeating and a bad diet can be matched by a spiritually bad diet and spiritual undernourishment. Both of these are highlighted by fasting which is capable of restoring the balance.

So it really depends upon us, we have the freedom to

choose a healthy diet benefiting body and soul. Fasting offers the chance of 'cleansing the inner man'.

The effects of fasting

Fasting is one of the most effective and natural treatments covering a wide range of disorders.
It works:
- in a preventive and in a healing way
- in curing disorders in the functioning of the body by:
- quick and safe weight loss
- breaking down sick, superfluous substance whilst preserving the healthy, properly functioning tissue
- reducing high blood pressure
- lessening the fat content of the blood
- adjusting the sugar count of the blood
- regulating the sedimentation in the body's blood
- relieving varicose veins
- improving the condition of intestinal and stomach passages
- restoring the gall bladder (even getting rid of small gall stones)

through
- the resulting loss of weight alleviating the spine and the joints of the body
- cleaning the body out leaving it free from poisons and various other residual matter
- easing the pancreas (to such an extent that some diabetics can manage without insulin during their fast and even after it as well)
- allowing the exchange of gases and substances to be made more easily
- increasing the strength of the heart and breathing (digestive activity decreases saving about 30% energy)

through
- diminishing arteriosclerotic deposits in the arteries

– destroying fat in the vascular wall

Fasting, therefore, presents itself as the ideal and most intensive treatment for the overweight with those accompanying symptoms and resultant diseases.

Because it has such wide-reaching effects on the general well-being of the patient, its compatibility and practicability together with its results make it much better than any alternative treatments.

Even in cases of 50% obesity in children, the majority of whom have been found to be about 13 years old, lasting weight losses have been obtained through fasting with no damaging effects. Normally, it should be said, children under 14 should not fast because it requires a decision taken freely and with understanding.

Fasting can be most beneficial before an operation as a preventative measure because:

– it leaves the patient in the best possible condition
– it increases the immunity of the blood against specific bacterial infections
– it thins the blood, reducing the dangers of thrombosis or heart attack
– the efficiency of the connective tissue is improved which is important in contributing to

> resistance to infection
> the formation of the blood
> the healing of wounds
> the formation of scar tissue

But the most important factor has to be the reduction in weight itself, particularly for orthopedic disorders, for most people with such problems are overweight. In consequence the static burden is too high and unless it is lightened even the best orthopedic operation will be ineffectual. In fact 'In many cases where the patient has lost weight the operation can either be postponed or avoided completely because associated pain will have diminished. This will be the case for about one in three patients.'

Apart from this fasting diminishes the risks involved with operations. It is particularly valuable to fast for 2–3 days drinking only fruit juice which prepares the stomach and intestines for the operation.

For which diseases can one and should one fast?

Fasting is recommended in cases of:
- heart and circulatory disorders
- stomach and intestine complaints
- diseases of the liver
- diseases of the kidneys
- kidney stones may pass out of the kidneys if they are not too big or be dissolved by the uric acid produced during a fast. 'Healing in its own way'
- diseases of the veins and skin

It can also be beneficial to fast in cases of:
- diabetes
- rheumatism of the joints or muscles
- degenerative diseases of the joints (less weight is always helpful, and according to which disease and its degree of seriousness another fast may be advisable)
- asthma improves with weight loss
- menopausal and menstruation problems
- chronic eye infections; fasting is particularly helpful used in conjunction with medication from an eye specialist.

The results of fasting include at the very least:
- a better general condition
- an improved performance and capacity to resist infection
- a better and younger appearance

Through a planned yearly fast you can preserve, or regain a better condition of the body; retain a healthy weight, or where necessary reduce it; and counter balance the damaging effects unavoidable in the environment.

Fasting and cancer prevention

Once cancer has been diagnosed it is usually treated by surgery, X-rays or chemotherapy. However, regular fasting is valuable as an important preventative factor against this disease.

At this point we should introduce the concept of a condition being 'precancerous'. That is, one which could be conducive to cancer; in this category one might include chronic infections or ulcers in the stomach or intestines. By fasting such disorders may be alleviated preventing the possibility of cancer.

The correlation between smoking and cancer is well known and it is apparent, for instance in the skin colour, that the body rids itself of more nicotine and tar while fasting. It is quite possible that this lowers the cancer risk, though it is, of course, essential to stop smoking altogether.

It is professionally agreed that 30–40% of terminal cancer cases are diet related particularly in cases where the disease attacks the oesophagus, stomach or large intestine. Our diet has increasingly included larger quantities of meat, sugar and especially fat while the roughage obtained from such things as wheat and potatoes has diminished. There are also cancer stimulating substances to be found in our modern environment and food. (*Prof Schmähl*, Cancer Research Centre, Heidelberg).

Those diseases which result from a bad diet and that could be precancerous should benefit particularly from fasting as a treatment.

Professor Dr Trüb an adviser to an association in Nordrheim-Westfalen fighting cancer, quotes the case of a female patient, very much overweight and at a precancerous stage in the condition of her reproductive organs who prevented cancer and slowed down the growth of existing swellings, by fasting. Both Dr Buchinger and his son have noted that cancer seldom afflicts those patients who year after year regularly fast as a preventive measure.

The German Cancer Congress in Munich observed that 'one of the greatest supports against cancer is the building up of our immunity strength'. It becomes more obvious from this what Dr Buchinger means when he declares that those forces existing in the body to fight disease are released by fasting.

> **When is fasting not recommended?**
> - in the case of all those diseases which destroy body
>   substances such as cancer, tuberculosis, bad neur-
>   oses and psychosis where all freewill has been closed
>   in
> - hysteria
> - when the elderly have lost too much weight
> - irrespective of age, when the body cannot respond
>   to the stimulation of a fast

It is quite reasonable to enquire if a fast can be damaging. But it is true to say that, when carried out correctly, fasting is easy and simple, and is almost universally recognised as an effective healing treatment. At the same time it is not a miracle-worker nor a cure-all, and there are cases where fasting is inadvisable and amongst these is cancer. Though, because of a lack of evidence, it is not really proven whether fasting might or might not be beneficial to cancer patients.

However, fasting is definitely not recommended in cases where the process of the disease destroys tissue which results in the loss of valuable body substances and cancer, particularly in its final stages, belongs in this category. Because conventional medicine is so limited in its ability to fight cancer experimenting with fasting is a possibility but only with a really competent cancer specialist.

Fasting is also inadvisable in cases where the body simply cannot respond to it positively. This might occur after a long debilitating illness that has resulted in the general weakening of the system or where there has been a considerable weight loss due to old age.

We should like to draw the attention of the reader to the fact that scientific research into fasting is far from complete. Also the highly complicated processes of the metabolism are still little known and the psychological ramifications of fasting have also yet to be fully understood. We can so far only recognise the cathartic effect, the mental cleansing process and the explanations acceptable in the field of psychic studies. The experiences of mystics and religious leaders give us an idea of the enormous possibilities in the spiritual field.

Whatever the circumstance of the question as to the

necessity for, or the meaning of, fasting it can be answered by Dr Buchinger's words 'fasting does no harm, and is always worth trying'.

After a fast

Those days following a fast are as important as the fast itself. It is as crucial to give yourself time at this stage as it is for the actual fast. The ideal situation would have as many days for 'building-up' as there are for fasting or at least a third to a half the time set aside for a fast should be used for adjusting back to food. The success of the fast can be put at risk if this building-up time is not adequately accounted for, it is necessary to sustain the result and it can even improve on it. If we take a fast of 3 weeks then from 7–15 days should be used for building-up.

The patient who is fasting must seriously consider the building-up time with equal attention. This involves introducing those food elements which are right for him after his fast a little at a time, of the correct quality and in the right quantity and mixture.

Fasting is easier than building up

The first few days after the fast are the most difficult to cope with.

They require great discipline, patience, caution and commonsense. For this reason it is necessary to:
- retain the relaxed, protected quietness and partial isolation which the fasting atmosphere provides
- keep away from stress as much as possible
- avoid returning to the burdens of professional and everyday life
- make no mistakes with food, by eating too much, or in between meals or having excess restaurant food
- continue abstaining from alcohol so as not to overload the liver again particularly when its tolerance level is still low.

Alcohol does not only damage the liver, which is central to the building-up process but hinders its function during this period of reintroducing food when there is so much for it to do. Adding alcohol can only make its job more difficult. Drinking alcohol and overeating just after a fast can not only produce slight but unpleasant digestive complaints but precipitate more serious, even dangerous consequences.

The feeling of hunger does not last long so the portions served are consequently small during the time just after a fast has ended. If you wish you can eat everything but you do not have to. As soon as you cease feeling hungry you should stop eating immediately. There should be no compulsion to make up for the meals missed while fasting. Even though a lot of food is puréed it is necessary to chew it conscientiously for each mouthful should be richly savoured. We are given the opportunity, which really must be taken, to concentrate completely on our food while we eat and we should not allow ourselves to be distracted by conversation.

It is advisable to take advantage of the time set aside for a rest before each meal but especially important to rest in bed after it. This ensures the digestive organs a good supply of blood which is more necessary now that the body has started to have food again. Physical exercise, however, would be wrong at this time.

After the fast, the fewer the rules (albeit important ones) to be followed together with the **continuation** of various therapies, the easier and better will be the transition back to normal life. It will:
- increase the production of digestive enzymes in accordance with their requirement
- initiate the first bowel movement as the intestines fill
- balance liquid retention, after the greater need of 1–2 litres is covered
- stimulate the circulation as the digestion requires it
- give the pains associated with past illness time to gradually disappear. These should never be considered dangerous or the result of a poor fast, they are a known factor of the 'after fast' phase.

A longer building-up period will be profitable for:
- training the patient into new eating habits

- getting to know a new, tastier and healthier meat-free diet
- avoiding those damaging foods and drinks like sweets, chocolates and alcohol, for longer and perhaps preventing their reintroduction into the diet
- gaining a new joyful dimension to life with a stronger resistance to disease
- losing even more weight if necessary
- consolidating the results already achieved.

Breaking a fast

This begins at midday with a fresh, ripe, unpeeled apple, a freshly grated apple or some apple purée. Apples are considered the best food with which to break a fast because of their taste, smell and pleasant fruit acids, they are also rich in pectin which is easy to digest and picks up poisons in the bowel. It is, however, very important to chew it well, remembering that digestion begins in the mouth. A second apple may be eaten in the afternoon.

In the evening vegetable or potato soup will be served either with no salt at all or perhaps, just a pinch of sea salt. At this meal the patient will receive his 'faster's diploma' which should make him conscious of beginning a new phase in his life for which he should be thankful. The table will be decorated with flowers and a candle to give the occasion a festive air.

Dr Buchinger said, 'Meals during the building-up period should be prepared without salt. This is because during the fast the patient will have lost a great deal of water from his body and ordinary salt helps retain water in the cells and would be harmful. If this rule is ignored the patient will suffer fatigue and eventually oedema. This results from drinking too much water because the salt makes him thirsty, this fills the cells and the space between them too quickly. This is a salutary lesson to the patient and may remind him that at least one of the most important rules of this building-up period must be adhered to.'

Building-up

Immediately after a fast the diet should be specially designed to contain foods rich in carbohydrates since they are the most compatible substances for the body. The addition of protein in the meals at this time could stimulate the unnecessary formation of gases because the digestive system has been inactive for such a long time.

The building-up diet

There are certain principles which should be followed when planning a diet for the building-up stage:
- it should consist as far as possible of natural products avoiding processed foods
- the food should be carefully prepared to avoid losing essential goodness (this would occur, for instance, if they are overheated or left in water for too long)
- it should exclude foods which cause or sustain fermentation, like white sugar and some processed foods
- it should contain foods that have a laxative effect to help bowel movement

Natural foods which have this effect contain the following elements:
- roughage or undigested cellulose, which by filling and therefore pushing against the intestinal walls act as stimulation to the peristaltic action of the intestines; this is found mostly in raw foods, salads, grains and fresh fruit
- natural acids; as with fruit acids, lactic acids and the natural fermentation in milk work a chemical stimulation on the peristalsis. So it is advisable to eat fruit, sour milk, yoghurt and sauerkraut and drink the juice of sauerkraut and celery
- lubricants – found in linseed, agar-agar, fats and oils. Such foods develop a strong mucosity under certain conditions which has a beneficial effect on the intestines.

Building-up menu

Here we offer some explanation concerning the meals served during the 'building-up' period.

Day 1

Breakfast – Apart from some dried prunes, which are easy to digest and act as a laxative, the patient will get some wheat bran purée. On this first day the bran is boiled having first been soaked overnight to prevent overworking the digestion.

Midday – Some raw vegetables or a salad should always be served at the beginning of a meal. They help to stimulate the digestive enzymes in the stomach as well as offering roughage, but more importantly they prevent the formation of digestive leukozytose. There will be included at this time food that activates the production of bile, however any sauce rich in oil will be counter-productive to this purpose. Fibrous vegetables such as spinach, fennel, asparagus and sauerkraut contain large amounts of roughage important to the intestines.

Evening – As an hors d'oeuvres exotic fruits like pineapple, melon and kiwi fruit are preferable. These fruits have a high enzyme content which in turn stimulates the enzymes of the body. A rice ring with cucumber and herbs is considered an easily digestible warm evening meal, and brown rice is particularly rich in minerals.

An apple is recommended as the last food of the day because it has both an alkaline effect and a cleansing effect on the intestines.

Day 2

Breakfast – On the second building-up day it is unnecessary to cook the wheat bran but it should be soaked and prepared like muesli.

Midday – A wheat soufflé made with raw grain is a particularly healthy meal because it contains necessary roughage and is most satisfying because the whole grains remain in the stomach for some time.

Evening – A mixture of curd and valuable vegetable oils gives the body important unsaturated vegetable fats.

Days 3 and 4

During the next 2 days variations on the foods already introduced will be served with specific and differing importance to the body.
- various grains   – a greater variety of raw foods
- more fats with rising calorific values

Building-up plan A

Breaking a fast: an apple or some apple purée, and in the
                 evening potato soup

Day 1

Breakfast: 2 prunes
                 some wheat mash with fig mousse, apple
                 and honey herb tea or malt coffee

10.00hrs: a natural yoghurt (in your room)

Midday: 1 portion of lettuce (chicory, radicchio, or
                 endive) potato purée and fresh spinach
                 with yeast extract

14.00 hrs: tea with lemon and a Buchinger vitamin
                 shake (in your room)

Dinner: 1 piece of fruit (melon, pineapple, or kiwi
                 fruit)
                 small portion of rice and cucumber with
                 herbs
                 tomato salad
                 herb tea or malt coffee

20.00 hrs: 1 apple

                              Nutritional value: 876 calories
                                 Protein 26 gr
                                 Fat 16 gr
                                 Carbohydrates 142 gr

Day 2

Breakfast:	2 prunes muesli with roasted almonds herb tea or malted coffee
10.00 hrs:	1 natural yoghurt (in your room)
Midday:	raw carrots, apples and nuts wheat soufflé grilled tomatoes with a tomato sauce
14.00 hrs:	tea with lemon and a Buchinger vitamin shake (in your room)
Dinner:	courgette salad baked potato with curd-oil cream garnished with 2 slices of egg
20.00 hrs:	1 apple (in your room)

> Nutritional value: 1069 calories
> Protein 44 gr
> Fat 31 gr
> Carbohydrates 135 gr

Day 3

Breakfast:	1 piece of fruit (melon, pineapple or kiwi fruit) museli with roasted almonds herb tea or malt coffee
10.00 hrs:	1 natural yoghurt (in your room)
Midday:	mixed salad with ground nuts omelette with a vegetable filling
14.00 hrs:	tea with lemon and a Buchinger vitamin shake (in your room)
Dinner:	celery leaf salad with walnuts millet paste with dill sauce vegetable paté 1 piece of hard corn bread herb tea or malt-coffee

20.00 hrs: 1 apple (in your room)

> Nutritional value: 1275 calories
> Protein 51 gr
> Fat 38 gr
> Carbohydrates 154 gr

Day 4

Breakfast: muesli with roasted almonds
1 piece of wholewheat bread
5 gr butter or margarine
50 gr curd cheese
15 gr honey
herb tea or malt coffee

10.00 hrs: 1 natural yoghurt (in your room)

Midday: salad with sesame seeds
vegetable flan with fresh mushrooms
and a light soya sauce
curd cheese with fruit and wheat grains

14.00 hrs: tea with lemon and a Buchinger vitamin
shake
(in your room)

Dinner: salad of lettuce with a yoghurt sauce
exotic soya ragout with curried rice
curd cream
5 gr butter or margarine
1 piece of hard corn bread
herb tea or malt coffee

20.00 hrs: 1 apple (in your room)

> Nutritional value: 1583 calories
> Protein 77 gr
> Fat 57 gr
> Carbohydrates 184 gr

Some of the main recipes used in the 'building-up' diet

Vegetable flan with mushrooms
Serves 3
384 calories per portion

Ingredients: for the flan:
5 oz or 150 gr wholemeat flour
1 egg
2½ oz or 60 gr vegetable oil magarine
1 tblsp each cider vinegar and water
pinch of herb salt

for the filling:
5 oz or 150 gr fresh mushrooms
5 oz or 150 gr celery
5 oz or 150 gr carrots
about 6 tblsp. skimmed milk
1 egg
½ oz or 10 gr yeast extract
2½ tblsp grated low fat cheese
2 tblsp fresh parsley
nutmeg, herb salt, vegetable stock

For the flan base; mix the ingredients together into a dough and roll it out. Place it into the greased flan dish to form a pastry case. For the filling; dice the vegetables and simmer for a few minutes in some water in a saucepan. Meanwhile whip the egg yolk, milk, yeast extract and seasoning to a creamy consistency. Beat the egg white until stiff then add it to the creamed mixture, then mix in the vegetables and put it all into the pastry case. Sprinkle the top with grated cheese and bake for 20 minutes at 350°F/180°C or Gas mark 4.

Millet paste with dill sauce
Serves 1
143 calories per portion

Ingredients: 1 oz or 20 gr cooked millet
½ tblsp small peas/petit pois
½ tblsp cooked, diced carrots
¼ egg
½ tblsp low fat curd cheese
fresh herbs and herb salt

Mix together the millet, peas and carrots. Then mix in the egg and curd cheese to make a paste adding a little water if necessary. Put the paste into a greased mould and allow it to set by placing in a basin of water.

Dill sauce: Take some of the stock left from cooking the vegetables and add an equal quantity of milk, mix in a little flour then add some sea salt and a generous amount of fresh dill and heat to allow the sauce to thicken.

Exotic Soya Ragout
Serves 2
85 calories per portion

Ingredients: 2 oz or 50 gr soya, already rehydrated
1 oz or 20 gr finely chopped onion
1 tblsp. raisins
1 oz or 10 gr beansprouts
Banana mousse, roughly grated pineapple
1 tblsp. thinly sliced mushrooms
1 cup of tomato juice

Simmer the onion in a little water; dice the soya, the raisins and beansprouts and add, with the mushrooms and pineapple to the onion. Simmer for a further 10 minutes. Top up the liquid with the tomato juice and season with banana mousse, honey, lemon juice and tamari or soya sauce.

Wheat Soufflé
Serves 1
171 calories per portion

Ingredients: 1 oz or 20 gr wheat
1 oz or 20 gr skimmed curd
¼ egg
¾ oz or 15 gr grated cheese
1 teasp oil for greasing dish
salt, pepper, herb salt, nutmeg, 1 drop tamari

Cook the wheat for a short time in some water. Let it cool then add the curd, egg, cheese and seasoning; mix well and turn into a greased baking dish. Either stand it in a basin of hot water or put in a moderate oven for 20 minutes to thicken.

Creamed curd for baked potatoes
Serves 1
104 calories per portion

Ingredients: 1 tblsp. skimmed curd mixed thoroughly with a little butter milk
2 teasp. oil (sunflower, linseed or thistle)
1 teasp. coarsely chopped sunflower seeds

Mix all the ingredients together and season with a little herb salt.

Coarsely-milled wheat roast
Serves 1
105 calories per portion

Ingredients: 1½ oz or 30 gr coarsely-milled wheat or rye
½ egg
1 teasp soya flour
1 teasp yeast extract
finely chopped parsley
sea salt and Vitamin R

Soak the grain overnight. Add to the softened grain all the other ingredients and mix well, season to taste then fry them in a very little oil.

Mushroom roast
Serves 2
157 calories per portion

Ingredients: 2 oz or 50 gr cooked mushrooms
1 egg
2 teasp soya flour
1 small grated onion
herb salt, lots of fresh herbs and Vitamin R

Mix all the ingredients together, season to taste then fry in a
very little oil.

Muesli

				Protein	Fat	Carbo-hydrates	Calories
1 teasp	10 gr	½ oz	Wheat	1.2	0.2	6.9	35
½ teasp	2 gr		Sunflower seeds	0.3	0.6	0.3	8
½ teasp	2 gr		Sesame seeds	0.4	1.0	0.4	12
1 teasp	1 gr		Linseeds	0.2	0.3	0.1	4
1 teasp	1 gr		Wheatgerm	0.3	0.1	0.5	4
½ teasp	1 gr		Raisins	+	−	0.6	3
	20 gr	1 oz	Skimmed curds	3.4	0.2	0.4	18
	60 gr	2½ oz	Apple	+	−	7.2	30
½ teasp	2 gr		Ground nuts	0.3	1.2	0.3	14
1 dsp	1 gr		Agar-agar	−	−	−	−
	2 gr		Soya milk powder	0.3	0.5	1.0	10
½ teasp	2 gr		Honey	+	−	1.6	6
	2 gr		Almonds	0.4	1.1	0.3	13
	2 gr		Lemon juice	+	−	0.2	1
	2 gr		Sea Buckthorn	+	−	1.2	5

In separate containers soak the wheat, sunflower seeds,
sesame seeds, linseeds and raisins in water overnight. In
the morning take the curds or yoghurt if preferred and mix
all the ingredients together with the exception of the
lemon juice and honey, and the apple. Grate the apple
freshly then add in lightly and season with the lemon juice
and honey just before serving.

Reasons for a vegetarian diet in the 'building-up' stage

A special building-up diet lasting for at least two weeks after the end of the fast has proved very successful in the many years we have used it. It completely excludes meat and fish and is recommended by the German Association for Nutrition. The diet is quite balanced because of its careful preparation and composition, and it contains:
- high value fats, carbohydrates and proteins
- vitamins
- flavour
- substances that stimulate fermentation
- auxins – growth promoting substances
- and minerals including potassium, calcium and magnesium which are known as bases.

These bases, which are generally found in vegetarian food and particularly in fruits such as lemons and in vegetables, neutralise the acids in meat, fish and cheese and most food originating from animals.

If there is insufficient of these bases in the diet, as seems prevalent in modern cooking with a predominance of meat, the body is forced to reach into the bones for it needs. This causes some decalcification and a loss of proteins with the formation of much residual matter in an attempt to maintain the important balance between the bases and acids.

It is essential that a healthy diet, rich in the bases, is maintained at all times but more particularly immediately after a fast. The proportion of potatoes, fruit and other vegetables should be from 5–7 times as great as the rest of the meal put together with some milk or milk products. It is important that a third of the raw and fresh fruit and vegetables with a corn mash be eaten at the beginning of the meal.

Processed foods should be avoided as much as possible. It is as well to change those foods that give what we call 'empty calories' or 'isolated carbohydrates' containing white flour and sugar for whole foods.

Animal fats should be replaced by vegetable oils and fats and the amount of salt reduced, but more fresh and dried herbs used instead.

It should be emphasised that less must be eaten; it is important to eat the right amount of the right food.

A diet high in calories containing a lot of meat, but with insufficient of the vital elements the body needs, leads to a great feeling of hunger and consequently a larger food intake meaning more stimulants. Compared with this, whole foods contain less protein resulting in fewer calories which cause a better performance from the body, better health and the capacity to reach and maintain a desirable weight.

In Germany 17 million DM are spent yearly in correcting the effects of what is termed the 'civilisation illnesses' caused by a harmfully rich diet. Having once fasted it is much easier to change from such a diet to a healthier one. Dr Buchinger said, 'That a patient who, having fasted, goes back to his old eating habits which may have caused him illness or weight problems, will soon lose the benefit of his fast and the better health it achieved for him.'

Examples of some fasts in relation to specific illnesses

Dr Buchinger's first experience with fasting himself was when he was completely cured of a severe rheumatic illness. In West Germany alone there are about 5.2 million rheumatism sufferers and of these 20,000 are declared invalids every year leaving them unable to work and the cost in social security benefits is very high.

Apart from this, fasting has an effect on illnesses related to our general metabolism and way of life. The problems of being overweight are often under-emphasised. For example the muscles of an overweight person need more oxygen than normal even when resting and this results in damaging the health of such an individual and threatening his life expectancy. At the same time the heart and circulatory system are overtaxed even before they are called upon for any extra exertion.

However, fasting is recommended for a person with no particular health problems as well, for in retrospect when studying a patient's medical history the benefits become apparent.

1. Fasting and muscular rheumatism

Mrs L. R. was 40 years old and overweight; she had some muscular heart problem, an overactive thyroid and some rheumatism with severe pain in her muscles. She embarked on a 50 day fast; on the 7th and 8th days she had a time of slight crisis but the inflammation slowly went and the pain disappeared. At the end of the fast her hands and upper arms were back to normal and the muscles and ligaments in her neck were relaxed and pain-free. An adjustment to a wholefood and vegetarian diet brought about a total change in the life of this patient.

2. Fasting and rheumatism of the joints (primal polyarthritis)

Mrs B. F. R. at 52 was 5 ft 6 in tall and weighed 9 st 2 lb. She had painful swelling of her knuckles, hands, elbows, shoulders and knees. She could not grasp anything with her hands nor bend or stretch her elbows and knees. After two introductory 'fruit days' she fasted for 41 days. She had a lot of pain and inflammation in her bad joints right up until the fifth week together with a high temperature and feverishness and could hardly move. However, in the sixth week a considerable change for the better occurred. Her temperature dropped and the periods of pain became fewer and less intense, the mobility increased in her joints and she could move about freely and then rest completely. Her fasting treatment was so successful that there was no need for her to return, as was expected, for a further fast 2 years later and today, 13 years afterwards, she lives a healthy problem-free life.

3. Rheumatoid arthritis

A 39 year old patient, suffering for 16 years from rheumatoid arthritis finally came for treatment in June 1971. During the previous years she had been in hospitals and sanatoriums on fifteen occasions and undergone cortisone treatment. When she arrived she weighed 6 st 2 lb and was 5 ft 11 in tall. To begin with she came off all the conventional medicines she was taking and was put onto a raw food diet. Her hand and knee joints were particularly badly inflamed and both shoulders and elbows were painful. She could move only with great difficulty and pain. Despite her low weight the patient began her fast. Though on the second and third days she had slight headaches and was sick several times, within a few days the pain began to diminish particularly in her shoulders and she could move her fingers and knees much better. Her weight went down to 5 st 11 lb by the 3rd day but she could almost clench her left hand. On the 7th day she had a high pulse rate and weighed only 5 st 8 lb but otherwise felt well. She continued fasting for 15 days being carefully monitored each day but while her weight dropped to 5 st 7 lb she began the building-up stage with no more pain, feeling very well and able to go back to work. Her weight went up to 5 st 11 lb and although she sometimes had slight pain still in her knees her general state of health was good. She later returned for a second fast and as a result has been without any pain since.

4. The effect of fasting on Rheumatoid arthritis

Mrs B. P. came from Folkestone, she was 52 years old, 5 ft 5½ in tall and weighed 11 st 6 lb. This particular patient had sought treatment for her severely and painfully inflamed joints in England, Baden Baden and South Africa. She had only found some relief after powerful cortisone treatment. When she arrived at the clinic she needed the help of two nurses as she could not travel or move about without assistance. She managed a 30 day fast only with the moral support of her husband and she had considerable pain all the time to start with. However, after 20 days of fasting the pain slowly began to recede and the patient managed to walk a little on the arm of her husband. She no longer used cortisone but turned to homoeopathic medicines. Her joints became more flexible, and her general state of health was improved, but when she left the clinic she was still in pain. She returned six months later to undergo another fast. On this occasion despite the pain and limited mobility she generally felt better. She fasted for 22 days and when she left the clinic this time she had almost no pain and no longer needed any medication and could manage to walk for up to about a mile and a half.

5. The effect of fasting on a blood clot in the artery of a leg

Mr E. M. came from Munich when he was 56 years old, he was 5 ft 10 in tall and weighed 12 st 14 lb. He had partial clotting in the artery of his left leg and found difficulty walking even short distances; this complaint is most common amongst smokers. Added to this he had recurrent angina pectoris and a high sugar count due very much to his age. The patient had been smoking 70 cigarettes a day and so before a fast could be contemplated he had to find a way to stop smoking. This was difficult but despite that the patient managed to give it up. After 2 introductory days on a diet he fasted for 27 days followed by an 11 day 'building-up' period. The absence of nicotine together with a well-planned programme of exercises proved most successful. In fact the surgeon who had been about to perform a complicated hip operation on this patient found it no longer necessary. In addition his sugar count was normal and he ceased to have heart problems.

6. The effect of fasting on inflammation of the kidneys

The history of kidney infections in an engineer who came to the clinic at the age of 49 started when he was only 6. As the result of an operation to remove his tonsils some time later he had a recurrence of this complaint. Then 2 years later after major dental treatment he successfully took a cure at Bad Bildungen. In 1957 he went on a fast for 21 days which proved so beneficial that he repeated it in 1960 and 1962. On the last two occasions his 14 day fasts included fruit and vegetable juices together with full massage and partial bath treatments. During these fasts he also took walks and went rowing, generally feeling that his performance was much improved and that his zest for life had grown. His blood pressure fell from 180/120 to 130/90 and laboratory tests that had for years shown poor health became normal. After one further fast it was shown from clinical tests that this patient was now quite well.

7. The effect of fasting on skin diseases

Mr F. M., 37 years old, 5 ft 10 in tall and weighing 13 st had suffered from discharging eczema all over his body. Hospital treatment on 2 occasions had been only moderately successful and so he had come to the clinic on the advice of his doctor. He underwent a 40 day fast with some homoeopathic treatment. In the 3rd week he reached a point of crisis when his abdomen and thighs became red and were discharging but after 4 days this passed. During the 5th and 6th weeks of his fast the patient found these symptoms disappeared and he left the clinic completely cured but with the strong recommendation that for a lasting effect he would have to change his diet.

8. The effect of fasting on obesity

Madame A. L. was aged 52 and weighed 15 st 9 lb, she had high blood pressure, palpitation, diabetes, a fatty liver and thromboses. She fasted for 21 days and as a result lost 19½ lb, her blood pressure fell from 185/110 to 145/90 and her cholesterol level from 259 to 163 and her sugar count from 199mg% to 72mg%. She stopped her medication, her heart and circulation became normal and the state of her blood pressure and her liver remained much improved.

9. The effect of fasting on diabetes

Mr J. F. weighed 18 st and was 5 ft 7½ in tall when he came for some fasting treatment at the age of 69. When he arrived he had diabetes and palpitations of the heart. He fasted for 18 days during which time he had no problems and lost 22 lb. His sugar count became normal and his heart complaint disappeared without need of medication.

10. The effect of fasting on liver disease

We had a 54 year old patient who was suffering from a chronically inflamed liver and the surface of whose skin was ulcerated. This man had been an alcoholic since his student days and had been treated by doctors one of whom finally recommended a fasting cure. On the first occasion he fasted for 14 days and followed it with a 'building-up' period. His condition improved, his laboratory tests were improved and the skin ulcers disappeared. The patient was conscious of feeling better and able to do much more. In the following years he returned for further fasting cures with the result that laboratory tests showed him fully recovered and he had no recurrence of the skin disease.

Where one can go to fast

GERMANY

Klinik Buchinger am Bodensee
Dr. med. Ch. Kuhn
Wilhelm-Beck-Straße 27
88662 Überlingen
Tel.: 0049-7551-8070

Klinik Dr. Otto Buchinger
Dr. med. Andreas Buchinger
Forstweg 39
31812 Bad Pyrmont
Tel.: 0049-5281-1660

Kurpark-Klinik
Dr. med. Gunther Hölz
Gällerstraße 10
88662 Überlingen
Tel.: 0049-7551-8060

Krankenhaus Moabit
Innere Abteilung (Naturheilweisen)
Professor Dr. M. Bühring
Dr. med. R. Stange
Turmstraße 21
10559 Berlin
Tel.: 0049-30-39760

Klinikum Berlin-Buch
Klinik für Physiotherapie
Dr. med. Jürgen Rohde
Wiltbergstraße 50
13125 Berlin
Tel.: 0049-30-94010

Klinik am Warteberg
Dr. med. Kai Sawatzki
Werner-Eisenberg-Weg 3
37213 Witzenhausen
Tel.: 0049-5542-5060

Schwarzwald-Sanatorium Obertal
Dr. med. Thomas Adrian
Rechtmurgstraße 27
72270 Baiersbronn-Obertal
Tel.: 0049-7449-840

Krankenhaus für Naturheilweisen
Sanatoriumsplatz 2
81545 München
Tel.: 0049-89-625050

Privatklinik Dr. Karl Spiske
Dr. med. Johann Hann
Bürgermeister-Ledermann-Straße 7
86819 Bad Wörishofen
Tel.: 0049-8247-3980

Klinik Dr. von Weckbecker
Dr. Erich von Weckbecker
Drs. Eva und Norbert Lischka
Rupprechtstraße 20
97769 Bad Brückenau
Tel.: 0049-9741-830

Birkle-Klinik
Dr. med. Tillo Soergel
Obere-St-Leonhard-Straße 55
88662 Überlingen
Tel.: 0049-7551-8030

AUSTRIA

Kur- und Gesundheitszentraum
Dr. Felbermayer
Dr. Michael Felbermayer
A-6793 Gaschurn/Montafon
Tel.: 0043-5558-8617

SWITZERLAND

LASSALLE-Haus Bad Schönbrunn
Pater Niklaus Brantschen SJ
CH-6313 Edlibach/Zug
Tel.: 0041-41-7571414

SPAIN

Clinica Buchinger S.A.
Frau Maria Buchinger
Herm Claus Rohrer
Dr. med. José-Manuel García-Verdugo
Apartado 68
E-29600 Marbella/Malaga
Tel.: 0034-5-276-4300
Fax: 0034-5-276-4305